LOW-FODMAP

FOOD LIST

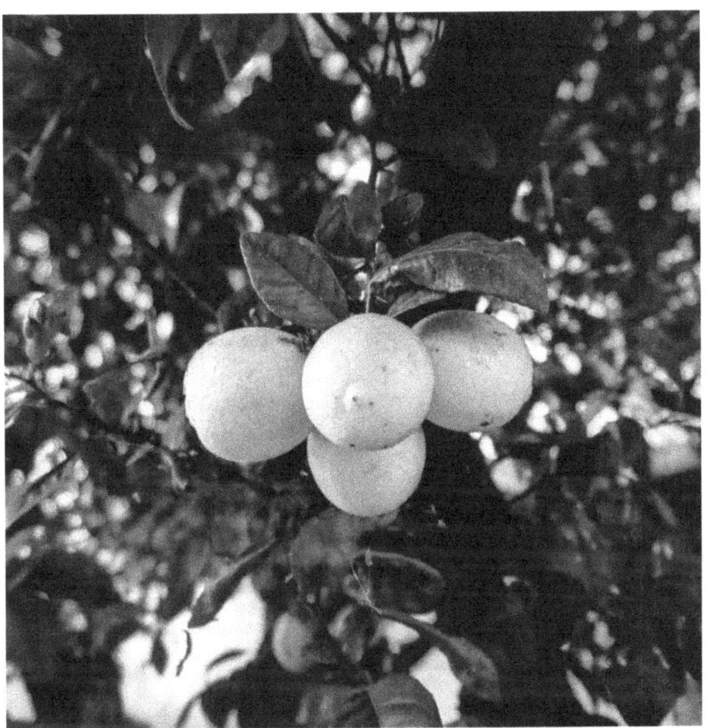

LORENE PEACHEY

DISCLAIMER

The content within this book reflects my thoughts, experiences, and beliefs. It is meant for informational and entertainment purposes. While I have taken great care to provide accurate information, I cannot guarantee the absolute correctness or applicability of the content to every individual or situation. Please consult with relevant professionals for advice specific to your needs.

TO GAIN ACCESS TO MORE BOOK BY THE AUTHOR SCAN THE QR CODE

TABLE OF CONTENTS

INTRODUCTION..1

CHAPTER 1...7

Understanding the Low FODMAP Diet 7

   What are FODMAPs? 7

   The Role of FODMAPs in Digestive Issues: 8

   Benefits of a Low FODMAP Diet: 9

CHAPTER 2 11

Identifying High and Low FODMAP Foods 11

   FODMAP Categories:... 11

   Reading Food Labels: 12

   Common High and Low FODMAP Foods: 13

CHAPTER 3 15

LOW-FODMAP Vegetables 15

CHAPTER 4 19

LOW FODMAP Fruits...19

CHAPTER 5 23

Grains and Cereals 23

CHAPTER 6 27

Proteins 27

CHAPTER 7 31

Dairy and Alternatives 31

CHAPTER 8 35

Herbs and Spices 35

CHAPTER 9 39

HIGH FODMAP FOOD TO AVOID OR LIMIT 39

CONCLUSION 43

BONUS CHAPTER 1 45

LOW-FODMAP RECIPES....................................45

BONUS CHAPTER 2 58

21 DAY MEAL PLAN...58

INTRODUCTION

In the enchanting world of nutrition, where the alchemy of flavors meets the science of well-being, I, Lorene Peachey, welcome you to a journey that has been the very essence of my life—a life devoted to unraveling the mysteries of dietary needs and crafting tantalizing recipes that not only nourish the body but also feed the soul.

As a seasoned nutritionist with over 25 years of experience, my quest for the perfect balance between health and indulgence has been nothing short of a culinary odyssey. Picture a kitchen filled with the rich aroma of wholesome ingredients, the sizzle of pans orchestrating a symphony of flavors, and the joyous laughter of those who have embraced the transformative power of mindful eating.

Have you ever wondered how the food we consume shapes not just our physical well-being but also our emotional and mental states? It's a profound question that has fueled my passion for nutritional research, and today, I invite you to explore this intricate relationship between what we eat and how we feel.

Imagine the sun-kissed glow of a summer morning as you take the first bite of a perfectly ripe peach, its juiciness trickling down your chin. That burst of sweetness isn't just a delightful flavor; it's a promise of a day filled with vitality. Now, contrast that with the heavy lethargy that follows a sugar-laden treat—like a fleeting spark that leaves you in the dark. Which scenario resonates with the life you want to lead?

In a world inundated with fast-paced living and convenience foods that often come at the cost of our well-being, I found myself asking a simple yet profound question: What if we could create a culinary symphony that not only delights our taste buds but also harmonizes with our body's intricate needs?

This question led me down a path of relentless research, a pursuit of uncovering the secrets hidden in the bounty of nature. As I delved deeper, it became clear that a low FODMAP approach to eating held the key—a key to unlocking a world of delicious possibilities for those seeking a healthier, happier life.

FODMAPs, short for Fermentable Oligosaccharides, Disaccharides, Monosaccharides, and Polyols, are a group of carbohydrates notorious for triggering digestive discomfort in susceptible individuals. Now, let me pose a question to you: How often have you found yourself plagued by the discomfort of bloating, gas, or stomach cramps, unknowingly imprisoned by the very foods that should nourish and sustain you?

In the pages of this book, I share with you not only the dangers and consequences of consuming high FODMAP foods but also the liberating magic of embracing a low FODMAP lifestyle. It's not just a dietary shift; it's a transformation—a journey toward reclaiming your digestive health and savoring the delights of a vibrant life.

As a nutritionist who has witnessed firsthand the transformative power of low FODMAP living, I can attest to the remarkable benefits it bestows upon those who choose this path. Imagine bidding farewell to the days of avoiding social gatherings or dreading meals because of the uncertainty of how your body will react. Picture a life where every bite is a celebration, and every meal is a step toward wellness.

The advantages of adopting a low FODMAP food list extend beyond the realms of digestive comfort. Say hello to increased energy levels, clearer skin, and a mind that is sharp and focused. Have you ever experienced the euphoria of feeling truly well—physically, mentally, and emotionally? It's a sensation that awaits you on this journey.

Now, let me share a secret with you—a secret that transcends the culinary realm and touches the very heart of our human experience. Food, my dear reader, is not merely sustenance; it's a language of love, a conduit for connection. How often have you sat around a table, sharing laughter and stories over a delightful meal? Food has the power to bring people together, to create memories that linger long after the plates are cleared.

In this book, I not only present you with a carefully curated low FODMAP food list but also with a treasury of recipes that elevate this journey from a dietary adjustment to a culinary celebration. From the tantalizing aroma of Grilled Lemon Herb Chicken to the comforting embrace of Quinoa Salad with Spinach and Feta, each recipe is a testament to the art of mindful cooking—a practice that transcends the boundaries of necessity and becomes a joyful expression of self-care.

Now, let's ponder another question together: What if you could turn your kitchen into a sanctuary—a place where the act of preparing a meal becomes a meditation, a moment of self-love? The low FODMAP food list presented in this book is not just a guide; it's an invitation to rediscover the joy of cooking and the pleasure of nourishing your body with intention.

As I stand at the crossroads of experience and innovation, I extend my hand to you, inviting you to embark on a transformative journey. This isn't just a book; it's a companion, a guide, and a celebration of the incredible potential that lies within the simple act of choosing what we put on our plates.

Together, let us turn the page to a life where every meal is a step toward vitality, where the joy of eating is matched only by the joy of living. Welcome to the world of low FODMAP living—a world where every bite is a declaration of self-love, and every recipe is a testament to the boundless possibilities that arise when we align our culinary choices with the rhythm of our bodies.

Join me as we explore the magic of low FODMAP cooking, where the simplicity of ingredients transforms into the symphony of a well-nourished life. Embrace this journey with open arms, dear reader, and let the pages that follow become your compass in the quest for a healthier, happier you.

Contact the Author

Thank you for reading my book! I would love to hear from you, whether you have feedback, questions, or just want to share your thoughts. Your feedback means a lot to me and helps me improve as a writer.

Please don't hesitate to reach out to me through

lorenepeachey@gmail.com

I look forward to connecting with my readers and appreciate your support in this literary journey. Your thoughts and comments are valuable to me.

CHAPTER 1

UNDERSTANDING THE LOW

FODMAP DIET

The Low FODMAP Diet has gained significant attention in recent years for its effectiveness in managing digestive issues. FODMAPs, or Fermentable Oligosaccharides, Disaccharides, Monosaccharides, and Polyols, are a group of short-chain carbohydrates that can trigger symptoms in individuals with certain digestive sensitivities. This Book will explore the nature of FODMAPs, their role in digestive issues, and the benefits associated with adopting a Low FODMAP Diet.

What are FODMAPs?

FODMAPs are a diverse group of carbohydrates found in various foods. The acronym stands for:

Fermentable: These carbohydrates are easily fermented by gut bacteria, leading to the production of gases.

Oligosaccharides: Complex carbohydrates such as fructans and galacto-oligosaccharides found in wheat, rye, onions, and legumes.

Disaccharides: Sugars like lactose, found in dairy products.

Monosaccharides: Single sugars, such as fructose, found in certain fruits like apples, honey, and high fructose corn syrup.

Polyols: Sugar alcohols found in some fruits and vegetables, as well as sugar substitutes like sorbitol and mannitol.

The Role of FODMAPs in Digestive Issues:

For individuals with certain digestive conditions like irritable bowel syndrome (IBS) and other functional gastrointestinal disorders, FODMAPs can contribute to symptoms such as bloating, gas, abdominal pain, and altered bowel habits. The presence of FODMAPs can draw water into the intestines and be fermented by gut bacteria, leading to the production of gas. In sensitive individuals, this can result in discomfort and exacerbate digestive symptoms.

Benefits of a Low FODMAP Diet:

Symptom Relief: The primary goal of adopting a Low FODMAP Diet is to alleviate symptoms associated with digestive disorders, particularly in individuals with IBS. By reducing the intake of high-FODMAP foods, many people experience a significant reduction in bloating, gas, and abdominal pain.

Improved Quality of Life: Managing digestive symptoms can enhance the overall quality of life for individuals with gastrointestinal disorders. The relief from daily discomfort allows for a more active and fulfilling lifestyle.

Identifying Trigger Foods: Following a Low FODMAP Diet involves a systematic elimination and reintroduction process. This helps individuals identify specific foods that trigger their symptoms, enabling them to make informed dietary choices and manage their condition more effectively.

Personalized Approach: The Low FODMAP Diet is not a one-size-fits-all solution. It can be tailored to individual tolerances and preferences. Working with a healthcare professional or a registered dietitian can help customize the diet to meet specific needs while ensuring nutritional adequacy.

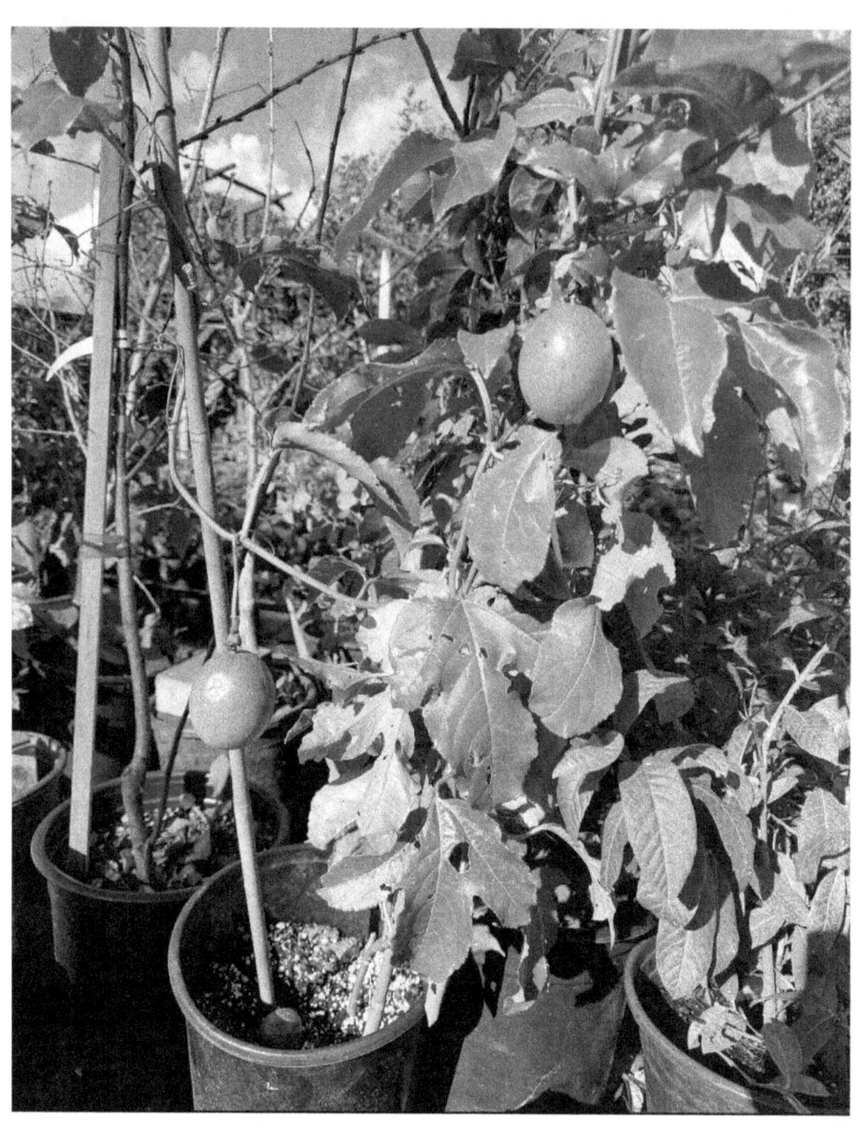

CHAPTER 2

IDENTIFYING HIGH AND LOW FODMAP FOODS

Successfully implementing a Low FODMAP Diet involves a thorough understanding of the FODMAP categories, the ability to read food labels, and knowledge of common high and low FODMAP foods. This article will guide you through these key aspects, helping you make informed choices to manage digestive symptoms effectively.

FODMAP Categories:

1. **Oligosaccharides:** Found in foods like wheat, rye, onions, garlic, and legumes.

2. **Disaccharides:** Present in dairy products containing lactose, such as milk, yogurt, and certain cheeses.

3. **Monosaccharides:** Include fruits like apples, pears, and honey, as well as foods with excess fructose, like high fructose corn syrup.

4. **Polyols:** Sugar alcohols found in certain fruits, vegetables, and artificial sweeteners like sorbitol and mannitol.

Reading Food Labels:

To identify and manage FODMAP intake, it's crucial to read food labels carefully. Look for terms related to FODMAPs, such as:

1. **Oligosaccharides:** Wheat, barley, rye, onions, garlic, and inulin (a type of fiber).

2. **Disaccharides:** Lactose, found in milk, yogurt, and some cheeses.

3. **Monosaccharides:** Fructose, often found in high fructose corn syrup, honey, and certain fruits.

4. **Polyols:** Sorbitol, mannitol, xylitol, and isomalt, commonly used as sugar substitutes.

Common High and Low FODMAP Foods:

High FODMAP Foods:

1. **Fruits:** Apples, pears, mangoes, cherries.

2. **Vegetables:** Onions, garlic, asparagus, mushrooms.

3. **Grains:** Wheat, rye, barley.

4. **Dairy:** Milk, yogurt, certain soft cheeses.

5. **Sweeteners:** Honey, high fructose corn syrup, certain sugar alcohols.

Low FODMAP Foods:

1. **Fruits:** Strawberries, blueberries, bananas, oranges.

2. **Vegetables:** Spinach, carrots, bell peppers, zucchini.

3. **Grains:** Quinoa, rice, oats (in moderate amounts).

4. **Dairy:** Lactose-free milk, hard cheeses.

5. **Sweeteners:** Maple syrup, stevia.

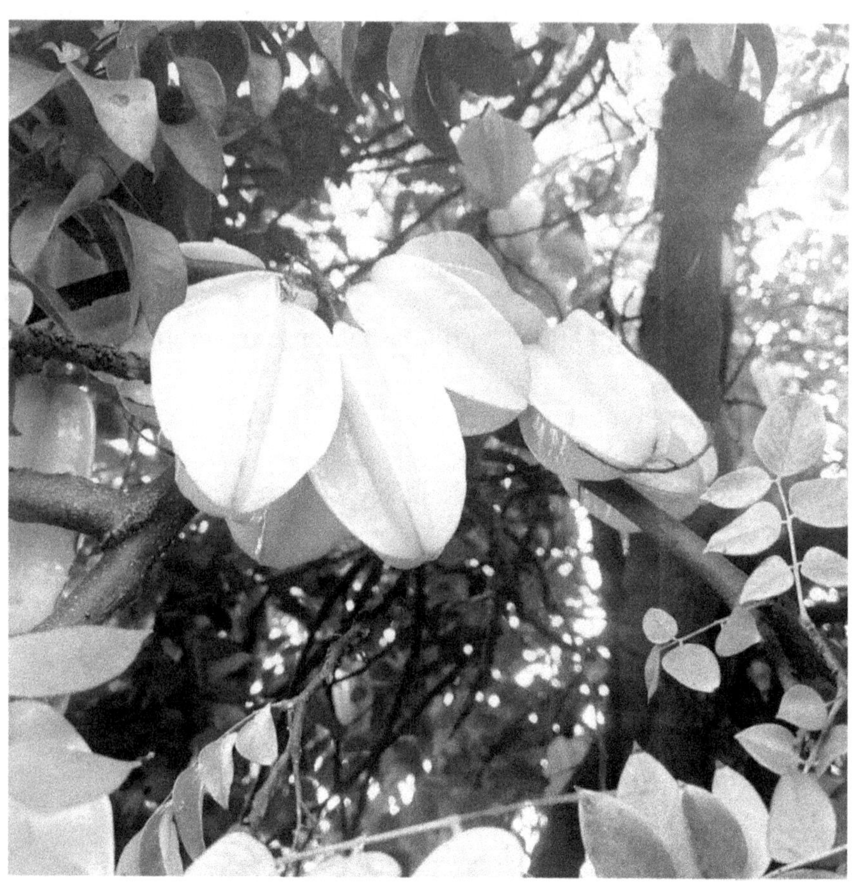

CHAPTER 3

LOW-FODMAP VEGETABLES

1. **Spinach:**

    - Serving Size: 1 cup (30g)

    - Calories: 7

    - Carbohydrates: 1g

    - Fiber: 1g

    - Protein: 1g

2. **Bell Peppers (Red):**

    - Serving Size: 1 medium pepper (186g)

    - Calories: 37

    - Carbohydrates: 9g

    - Fiber: 3g

    - Protein: 1g

3. **Carrots:**

- Serving Size: 1 medium carrot (61g)

- Calories: 25

- Carbohydrates: 6g

- Fiber: 2g

- Protein: 0.5g

4. **Zucchini:**

- Serving Size: 1 medium zucchini (196g)

- Calories: 33

- Carbohydrates: 6g

- Fiber: 2g

- Protein: 2g

5. **Cucumbers:**

- Serving Size: 1 cup sliced (133g)

- Calories: 16

- Carbohydrates: 4g

- Fiber: 1g

- Protein: 1g

6. **Tomatoes:**

- Serving Size: 1 medium tomato (123g)
- Calories: 22
- Carbohydrates: 5g
- Fiber: 2g
- Protein: 1g

7. **Green Beans:**

- Serving Size: 1 cup (100g)
- Calories: 31
- Carbohydrates: 7g
- Fiber: 3g
- Protein: 2g

8. **Eggplant:**

- Serving Size: 1 cup cubes (82g)
- Calories: 20
- Carbohydrates: 5g
- Fiber: 3g
- Protein: 1g

9. **Bok Choy:**

- Serving Size: 1 cup shredded (70g)

- Calories: 9

- Carbohydrates: 1g

- Fiber: 1g

- Protein: 1g

10. **Lettuce (Romaine):**

- Serving Size: 1 cup shredded (47g)

- Calories: 8

- Carbohydrates: 2g

- Fiber: 1g

- Protein: 1g

CHAPTER 4

LOW FODMAP FRUITS

1. **Limes:**

    - Serving Size: 1 medium lime (67g)

    - Calories: 20

    - Carbohydrates: 7g

    - Fiber: 2g

    - Protein: 1g

2. **Papaya:**

    - Serving Size: 1 cup cubes (140g)

    - Calories: 59

    - Carbohydrates: 15g

    - Fiber: 3g

    - Protein: 1g

3. **Passionfruit:**

- Serving Size: 1 medium passionfruit (18g)

- Calories: 17

- Carbohydrates: 4g

- Fiber: 3g

- Protein: 1g

4. **Starfruit:**

- Serving Size: 1 medium starfruit (196g)

- Calories: 45

- Carbohydrates: 11g

- Fiber: 3g

- Protein: 2g

5. **Blueberries:**

- Serving Size: 1 cup (148g)

- Calories: 84

- Carbohydrates: 21g

- Fiber: 4g

- Protein: 1g

6. **Bananas:**

- Serving Size: 1 medium banana (118g)

- Calories: 105

- Carbohydrates: 27g

- Fiber: 3g

- Protein: 1g

7. **Oranges:**

- Serving Size: 1 medium orange (131g)

- Calories: 62

- Carbohydrates: 15g

- Fiber: 3g

- Protein: 1g

8. **Kiwi:**

- Serving Size: 1 medium kiwi (100g)

- Calories: 61

- Carbohydrates: 15g

- Fiber: 3g

- Protein: 1g

9. **Raspberry:**

- Serving Size: 1 cup (123g)

- Calories: 65

- Carbohydrates: 15g

- Fiber: 8g

- Protein: 1g

10. **Honeydew Melon:**

- Serving Size: 1 cup cubes (177g)

- Calories: 64

- Carbohydrates: 16g

- Fiber: 1g

- Protein: 1g

CHAPTER 5

GRAINS AND CEREALS

1. **Quinoa:**

   - Serving Size: 1 cup cooked (185g)

   - Calories: 222

   - Carbohydrates: 39g

   - Fiber: 5g

   - Protein: 8g

2. **Rice (white):**

   - Serving Size: 1 cup cooked (195g)

   - Calories: 205

   - Carbohydrates: 45g

   - Fiber: 1g

   - Protein: 4g

3. **Oats (certified gluten-free):**

- Serving Size: 1 cup cooked (234g)

- Calories: 154

- Carbohydrates: 27g

- Fiber: 4g

- Protein: 6g

4. **Polenta:**

- Serving Size: 1 cup cooked (160g)

- Calories: 150

- Carbohydrates: 32g

- Fiber: 2g

- Protein: 3g

5. **Cornflakes (gluten-free):**

- Serving Size: 1 cup (28g)

- Calories: 100

- Carbohydrates: 24g

- Fiber: 0g

- Protein: 1g

6. **Buckwheat:**

- Serving Size: 1 cup cooked (168g)

- Calories: 155

- Carbohydrates: 33g

- Fiber: 5g

- Protein: 6g

7. **Millet:**

- Serving Size: 1 cup cooked (174g)

- Calories: 207

- Carbohydrates: 41g

- Fiber: 2g

- Protein: 6g

8. **Sorghum:**

- Serving Size: 1 cup cooked (192g)

- Calories: 220

- Carbohydrates: 48g

- Fiber: 6g

- Protein: 10g

9. **Rice Noodles (gluten-free):**

- Serving Size: 1 cup cooked (158g)

- Calories: 192

- Carbohydrates: 43g

- Fiber: 1g

- Protein: 4g

10. **Amaranth:**

- Serving Size: 1 cup cooked (246g)

- Calories: 251

- Carbohydrates: 46g

- Fiber: 5g

- Protein: 9g

CHAPTER 6

PROTEINS

1. **Chicken Breast (skinless, grilled):**

    - Serving Size: 3 ounces (85g)

    - Calories: 120

    - Protein: 26g

    - Fat: 2.5g

    - Carbohydrates: 0g

2. **Turkey (ground, cooked):**

    - Serving Size: 3 ounces (85g)

    - Calories: 135

    - Protein: 22g

    - Fat: 5g

    - Carbohydrates: 0g

3. **Fish (Salmon, baked):**

- Serving Size: 3 ounces (85g)

- Calories: 175

- Protein: 22g

- Fat: 9g

- Carbohydrates: 0g

4. **Tofu:**

- Serving Size: 1/2 cup (126g)

- Calories: 94

- Protein: 10g

- Fat: 6g

- Carbohydrates: 3g

5. **Eggs (boiled):**

- Serving Size: 2 large eggs (100g)

- Calories: 140

- Protein: 12g

- Fat: 9g

- Carbohydrates: 1g

6. **Shrimp (boiled or grilled):**

- Serving Size: 3 ounces (85g)

- Calories: 84

- Protein: 18g

- Fat: 1g

- Carbohydrates: 0g

7. **Lamb (chops, grilled):**

- Serving Size: 3 ounces (85g)

- Calories: 204

- Protein: 23g

- Fat: 12g

- Carbohydrates: 0g

8. **Pork (tenderloin, roasted):**

- Serving Size: 3 ounces (85g)

- Calories: 122

- Protein: 22g

- Fat: 3g

- Carbohydrates: 0g

9. **Firm Tofu:**

- Serving Size: 1/2 cup (126g)

- Calories: 94

- Protein: 10g

- Fat: 6g

- Carbohydrates: 3g

10. **Canned Tuna (in water):**

- Serving Size: 3 ounces (85g)

- Calories: 99

- Protein: 22g

- Fat: 1g

- Carbohydrates: 0g

CHAPTER 7

DAIRY AND ALTERNATIVES

1. **Lactose-Free Milk (e.g., lactose-free cow's milk or almond milk):**

   - Serving Size: 1 cup (240ml)

   - Calories: 80

   - Protein: 1g

   - Fat: 3g

   - Carbohydrates: 13g

2. **Feta Cheese (lactose-free or aged):**

   - Serving Size: 1 ounce (28g)

   - Calories: 74

   - Protein: 4g

   - Fat: 6g

   - Carbohydrates: 1g

3. **Hard Cheese (Cheddar, Swiss, Parmesan):**

- Serving Size: 1 ounce (28g)

- Calories: 110

- Protein: 7g

- Fat: 9g

- Carbohydrates: 0g

4. **Greek Yogurt (lactose-free or low-lactose):**

- Serving Size: 1 cup (227g)

- Calories: 120

- Protein: 20g

- Fat: 0g

- Carbohydrates: 10g

5. **Butter (lactose-free or clarified):**

- Serving Size: 1 tablespoon (14g)

- Calories: 102

- Protein: 0g

- Fat: 12g

- Carbohydrates: 0g

6. **Almond Milk (unsweetened, low FODMAP):**

- Serving Size: 1 cup (240ml)

- Calories: 30

- Protein: 1g

- Fat: 2.5g

- Carbohydrates: 1g

7. **Coconut Milk (canned, unsweetened):**

- Serving Size: 1 cup (240ml)

- Calories: 50

- Protein: 1g

- Fat: 5g

- Carbohydrates: 1g

8. **Brie Cheese:**

- Serving Size: 1 ounce (28g)

- Calories: 94

- Protein: 6g

- Fat: 8g

- Carbohydrates: 0g

9. **Lactose-Free Cottage Cheese:**

- Serving Size: 1 cup (240g)

- Calories: 210

- Protein: 28g

- Fat: 8g

- Carbohydrates: 6g

10. **Soy Milk (unsweetened, low FODMAP):**

- Serving Size: 1 cup (240ml)

- Calories: 80

- Protein: 7g

- Fat: 4g

- Carbohydrates: 4g

CHAPTER 8

HERBS AND SPICES

1. **Basil (Fresh):**

   - Serving Size: 2 tablespoons (5g)

   - Calories: 2

   - Carbohydrates: 0.4g

   - Fiber: 0.3g

   - Protein: 0.2g

2. **Chives (Fresh):**

   - Serving Size: 1 tablespoon (3g)

   - Calories: 1

   - Carbohydrates: 0.2g

   - Fiber: 0.1g

   - Protein: 0.1g

3. **Coriander (Ground):**

- Serving Size: 1 tablespoon (5g)

- Calories: 15

- Carbohydrates: 2.8g

- Fiber: 2.1g

- Protein: 0.6g

4. **Dill (Fresh):**

- Serving Size: 1 tablespoon (3g)

- Calories: 0

- Carbohydrates: 0g

- Fiber: 0g

- Protein: 0g

5. **Ginger (Ground):**

- Serving Size: 1 teaspoon (2g)

- Calories: 6

- Carbohydrates: 1.4g

- Fiber: 0.2g

- Protein: 0.1g

6. **Parsley (Fresh):**

- Serving Size: 2 tablespoons (8g)

- Calories: 2

- Carbohydrates: 0.3g

- Fiber: 0.2g

- Protein: 0.2g

7. **Rosemary (Dried):**

- Serving Size: 1 teaspoon (1g)

- Calories: 2

- Carbohydrates: 0.5g

- Fiber: 0.3g

- Protein: 0.1g

8. **Thyme (Fresh):**

- Serving Size: 1 tablespoon (2g)

- Calories: 2

- Carbohydrates: 0.5g

- Fiber: 0.3g

- Protein: 0.1g

9. **Turmeric (Ground):**

- Serving Size: 1 teaspoon (2g)

- Calories: 8

- Carbohydrates: 1.4g

- Fiber: 0.3g

- Protein: 0.2g

10. **Cumin (Ground):**

- Serving Size: 1 teaspoon (2g)

- Calories: 8

- Carbohydrates: 1.3g

- Fiber: 0.2g

- Protein: 0.3g

CHAPTER 9

HIGH FODMAP FOOD TO AVOID

OR LIMIT

1. **Wheat-based products (e.g., bread, pasta, and cereals):**

    - Serving Size: 1 slice of bread (25g)

    - Calories: 65

    - Carbohydrates: 12g

    - Fiber: 1g

    - Protein: 2g

2. **Onions:**

    - Serving Size: 1 medium onion (110g)

    - Calories: 44

    - Carbohydrates: 10g

    - Fiber: 2g

    - Protein: 1g

3. **Garlic:**

- Serving Size: 1 clove (3g)

- Calories: 4

- Carbohydrates: 1g

- Fiber: 0g

- Protein: 0g

4. **Milk (high lactose content):**

- Serving Size: 1 cup (240ml)

- Calories: 103

- Carbohydrates: 12g

- Fiber: 0g

- Protein: 8g

5. **Apples:**

- Serving Size: 1 medium apple (182g)

- Calories: 95

- Carbohydrates: 25g

- Fiber: 4g

- Protein: 0g

6. **Pears:**

- Serving Size: 1 medium pear (178g)

- Calories: 101

- Carbohydrates: 27g

- Fiber: 6g

- Protein: 1g

7. **Honey:**

- Serving Size: 1 tablespoon (21g)

- Calories: 64

- Carbohydrates: 17g

- Fiber: 0g

- Protein: 0g

8. **Cauliflower:**

- Serving Size: 1 cup chopped (100g)

- Calories: 25

- Carbohydrates: 5g

- Fiber: 3g

- Protein: 2g

9. **Watermelon:**

- Serving Size: 1 cup diced (152g)

- Calories: 46

- Carbohydrates: 12g

- Fiber: 1g

- Protein: 1g

10. **Beans (e.g., chickpeas, lentils):**

- Serving Size: 1 cup cooked (198g)

- Calories: 230

- Carbohydrates: 40g

- Fiber: 15g

- Protein: 15g

CONCLUSION

As we reach the final chapter of this culinary voyage, my heart swells with gratitude and anticipation. Together, we've uncovered the transformative power of low FODMAP living—a journey not just about food but about reclaiming our joy, vitality, and connection to the world around us.

As you embark on this new chapter of your culinary adventure, armed with a low FODMAP food list and a treasure trove of delectable recipes, I invite you to savor every moment. Let the kitchen become your sanctuary, a space where you craft not just meals but moments of love and well-being.

Remember, this isn't a farewell; it's a commencement—a commencement of a life where your relationship with food is a harmonious dance, where each ingredient is a partner in your well-being. The joy that emanates from mindful cooking is an everlasting gift—one that unfolds with each beautifully prepared dish and resonates in the shared laughter around your dining table.

But our journey doesn't end here; it merely takes on a new form. I invite you to share your experiences, your discoveries, and your own culinary creations. Your feedback is the heartbeat of this journey, and I eagerly anticipate hearing your stories of triumph, of moments where a simple recipe became a source of comfort or celebration.

Let this book be a conversation—a dialogue between us, between you and the recipes, between your well-being and the food you choose. Your voice matters, and your insights can inspire not just me but others on a similar path.

As you close this book, may you carry with you the flavors of joy, the aromas of self-care, and the knowledge that you hold the power to transform your life—one delicious bite at a time. Thank you for allowing me to be a part of your culinary expedition. Here's to a future filled with health, happiness, and the boundless possibilities that await in the kitchen of your dreams.

Cheers to you, to your journey, and to the countless meals that await your tender touch and creative spirit. Until we meet again, keep savoring the magic of mindful cooking, and may each meal be a celebration of the vibrant life you deserve. Bon appétit, dear friend!

BONUS CHAPTER 1

LOW-FODMAP RECIPES

Grilled Lemon Herb Chicken

- **Cooking Time:** 25 minutes

- **Servings:** 4

Ingredients:

- 4 boneless, skinless chicken breasts

- 2 tablespoons olive oil

- 1 lemon (juiced)

- 2 tablespoons fresh basil (chopped)

- Salt and pepper to taste

Instructions:

1. Preheat your grill to medium-high heat.

2. In a small bowl, mix together olive oil, lemon juice, chopped basil, salt, and pepper.

3. Place the chicken breasts in a resealable plastic bag and pour half of the marinade over them. Seal the bag and let it marinate in the refrigerator for 15 minutes.

4. Remove chicken from the bag and discard the used marinade.

5. Grill the chicken for 6-8 minutes per side or until fully cooked.

6. Drizzle the remaining marinade over the grilled chicken before serving.

Nutritional Information: Calories: 250, Protein: 30g, Carbohydrates: 1g, Fat: 14g, Fiber: 0g

Quinoa Salad with Spinach and Feta

- **Cooking Time:** 20 minutes

- **Servings:** 6

Ingredients:

- 2 cups cooked quinoa

- 2 cups fresh spinach

- 1/2 cup feta cheese (crumbled)

- 1/4 cup pine nuts

- 2 tablespoons olive oil

Instructions:

1. In a large bowl, combine the cooked quinoa, fresh spinach, crumbled feta, and pine nuts.

2. Drizzle olive oil over the mixture and toss until everything is evenly coated.

3. Season with salt and pepper to taste.

4. Serve chilled.

Nutritional Information: Calories: 220, Protein: 8g, Carbohydrates: 18g, Fat: 14g, Fiber: 3g

Baked Salmon with Lemon and Dill

- **Cooking Time:** 15 minutes

- **Servings:** 2

Ingredients:

- 2 salmon fillets

- 1 lemon (sliced)

- 2 tablespoons fresh dill (chopped)

Instructions:

1. Preheat your oven to 400°F (200°C).

2. Place the salmon fillets on a baking sheet lined with parchment paper.

3. Season the salmon with salt and pepper to taste.

4. Arrange lemon slices on top of the salmon and sprinkle with chopped dill.

5. Bake for 12-15 minutes or until the salmon is cooked through.

6. Serve with additional lemon wedges if desired.

Nutritional Information: Calories: 300, Protein: 30g, Carbohydrates: 1g, Fat: 20g, Fiber: 0g

Zucchini Noodles with Pesto

- **Cooking Time:** 15 minutes

- **Servings:** 4

Ingredients:

- 4 medium zucchinis (spiralized)

- 1/2 cup homemade or store-bought low FODMAP pesto

- 1/4 cup grated Parmesan cheese

- Salt and pepper to taste

Instructions:

1. Spiralize the zucchinis into noodles.

2. In a large pan, heat the pesto over medium heat.

3. Add the zucchini noodles to the pan and sauté for 5 minutes, or until they are just tender.

4. Season with salt and pepper to taste.

5. Serve the zucchini noodles topped with grated Parmesan cheese.

Nutritional Information: Calories: 150, Protein: 5g, Carbohydrates: 8g, Fat: 12g, Fiber: 3g

Turkey and Vegetable Skewers

- **Cooking Time:** 20 minutes

- **Servings:** 4

Ingredients:

- 1 pound ground turkey

- 1 zucchini, cut into chunks

- 1 red bell pepper, cut into chunks

- 1 tablespoon olive oil

- 1 teaspoon dried oregano

Instructions:

1. Preheat your grill or grill pan over medium-high heat.

2. In a bowl, mix ground turkey, olive oil, dried oregano, salt, and pepper.

3. Form the turkey mixture into small balls and thread them onto skewers alternately with zucchini and red bell pepper chunks.

4. Grill the skewers for 8-10 minutes, turning occasionally, until the turkey is cooked through and the vegetables are tender.

5. Serve the skewers hot.

Nutritional Information: Calories: 280, Protein: 25g, Carbohydrates: 5g, Fat: 18g, Fiber: 2g

Grilled Shrimp and Vegetable Skewers

- **Cooking Time:** 15 minutes

- **Servings:** 4

Ingredients:

- 1 pound large shrimp, peeled and deveined

- 1 zucchini, cut into chunks

- 1 yellow bell pepper, cut into chunks

- 1 tablespoon olive oil

- 2 tablespoons fresh parsley (chopped)

- Lemon wedges for serving

Instructions:

1. Preheat your grill to medium-high heat.

2. In a bowl, toss shrimp, zucchini, and bell pepper with olive oil, chopped parsley, salt, and pepper.

3. Thread the shrimp and vegetables onto skewers.

4. Grill for 3-4 minutes per side or until shrimp are opaque.

5. Serve with lemon wedges.

Nutritional Information: Calories: 180, Protein: 22g, Carbohydrates: 5g, Fat: 8g, Fiber: 2g

Eggplant Parmesan

- **Cooking Time:** 40 minutes

- **Servings:** 4

Ingredients:

- 1 large eggplant, sliced into rounds

- 1 cup lactose-free mozzarella cheese (shredded)

- 1 cup low FODMAP marinara sauce

- 1/2 cup Parmesan cheese (grated)

- 2 tablespoons fresh basil (chopped)

Instructions:

1. Preheat your oven to 375°F (190°C).

2. Lay eggplant slices on a baking sheet and sprinkle with salt. Let them sit for 15 minutes, then pat dry.

3. In a greased baking dish, layer eggplant slices, marinara sauce, mozzarella, and Parmesan cheese.

4. Repeat the layers and finish with a sprinkle of chopped basil.

5. Bake for 25-30 minutes or until bubbly and golden brown.

Nutritional Information: Calories: 250, Protein: 15g, Carbohydrates: 15g, Fat: 14g, Fiber: 5g

Lemon Herb Salmon with Quinoa

- **Cooking Time:** 25 minutes

- **Servings:** 4

Ingredients:

- 4 salmon fillets

- 1 cup quinoa (cooked)

- 2 tablespoons fresh dill (chopped)

- 1 lemon (zested and juiced)

- 2 tablespoons olive oil

Instructions:

1. Preheat your oven to 400°F (200°C).

2. Place salmon fillets on a baking sheet lined with parchment paper.

3. In a bowl, mix chopped dill, lemon zest, lemon juice, olive oil, salt, and pepper.

4. Brush the salmon with the lemon herb mixture.

5. Bake for 15-18 minutes or until salmon is cooked through.

6. Serve over a bed of cooked quinoa.

Nutritional Information: Calories: 350, Protein: 30g, Carbohydrates: 20g, Fat: 15g, Fiber: 3g

Chicken and Vegetable Stir-Fry

- **Cooking Time:** 20 minutes

- **Servings:** 4

Ingredients:

- 1 pound boneless, skinless chicken breast (sliced)

- 2 cups broccoli florets

- 1 red bell pepper (sliced)

- 1 carrot (julienne)

- 2 tablespoons low FODMAP stir-fry sauce

- 2 tablespoons sesame oil

- Green onions (green parts only) for garnish

- Cooked rice for serving

Instructions:

1. In a wok or large skillet, heat sesame oil over medium-high heat.

2. Add sliced chicken and cook until browned and cooked through.

3. Add broccoli, bell pepper, and carrot to the wok. Stir-fry for 3-4 minutes.

4. Pour in the stir-fry sauce and toss until everything is coated and heated through.

5. Serve over cooked rice and garnish with green onions.

Nutritional Information: Calories: 300, Protein: 25g, Carbohydrates: 20g, Fat: 12g, Fiber: 4g

Low FODMAP Caprese Salad

- **Cooking Time:** 10 minutes

- **Servings:** 2

Ingredients:

- 2 medium-sized tomatoes (sliced)

- 1 cup lactose-free mozzarella cheese (sliced)

- Fresh basil leaves

- 2 tablespoons extra-virgin olive oil

- Balsamic glaze for drizzling

- Salt and pepper to taste

Instructions:

1. Arrange tomato and mozzarella slices on a serving platter.

2. Tuck fresh basil leaves between the slices.

3. Drizzle with extra-virgin olive oil and balsamic glaze.

4. Season with salt and pepper to taste.

5. Serve immediately.

Nutritional Information: Calories: 250, Protein: 12g, Carbohydrates: 6g, Fat: 20g, Fiber: 2g

IF YOU WANT MORE RECIPES, YOU CAN CHECK OUT

OTHER BOOKS BY THE AUTHOR

GLUTEN-FREE COOKBOOK FOR MEN

GLUTEN-FREE SLOW COOKER COOKBOOK

TYPE 2 DIABETES INSTANT POT COOKBOOK

MEDITERRANEAN DIET COOKBOOK FOR NEWBIES

2024

GLUTEN-FREE AIR FRYER COOKBOOK

TO GET ACCESS TO MORE BOOKS BY THE AUTHOR

SCAN THE QR CODE

BONUS CHAPTER 2

21 DAY MEAL PLAN

Day	Breakfast	Lunch	Dinner	Snack
1	Scrambled Eggs with Spinach	Grilled Chicken Salad	Quinoa with Grilled Salmon	Carrot Sticks with Lactose-Free Cheese
2	Overnight Oats with Blueberries	Turkey and Veggie Wrap	Baked Chicken with Roasted Carrots	Strawberries with lactose-free Yogurt
3	Smoothie with Banana (ripe)	Zucchini Noodles with Pesto	Stir-Fried Shrimp with Rice	Rice Cakes with Almond Butter
4	Lactose-Free Yogurt with Kiwi	Caprese Salad	Turkey and Vegetable Skewers	Mixed Nuts

5	Omelette with Tomatoes	Quinoa Salad with Grilled Shrimp	Eggplant Parmesan	Grapes
6	Chia Seed Pudding with Banana	Chicken and Vegetable Stir-Fry	Grilled Lemon Herb Chicken	Lactose-Free Cheese Cubes
7	Pancakes with Maple Syrup	Tuna Salad with Leafy Greens	Baked Cod with Lemon and Dill	Orange Slices
8	Greek Yogurt Parfait	Low FODMAP Veggie Burger	Pork Tenderloin with Green Beans	Rice Crackers with Tuna Salad
9	Smoothie Bowl with Strawberries	Quinoa Stuffed Bell Peppers	Shrimp and Zucchini Stir-Fry	Mixed Berries with Almond Milk
10	Lactose-Free Cottage	Chicken Caesar Salad	Grilled Turkey with Sweet	Cucumber Slices with Hummus

	Cheese with Pineapple		Potato Wedges	
11	FODMAP-Friendly Muffins	Salmon and Spinach Salad	Quinoa Risotto with Asparagus	Rice Cakes with Peanut Butter
12	Frittata with Tomatoes and Feta	Turkey and Cranberry Wrap	Baked Ziti with Lactose-Free Cheese	Cherry Tomatoes with Balsamic Glaze
13	Banana (unripe) with Almond Butter	Grilled Veggie Bowl	Lemon Herb Tofu Skewers	Popcorn with Olive Oil
14	Low FODMAP Smoothie	Shrimp and Avocado Salad	Beef Stir-Fry with Broccoli	Pineapple Chunks
15	Quinoa Porridge with Strawberries	Turkey Lettuce Wraps	Grilled Lamb Chops	Carrot and Cucumber Sticks with Hummus

			with Quinoa	
16	Rice Cake with Lactose-Free Cream Cheese	Caprese Sandwich	Baked Salmon with Herbed Potatoes	Blueberries with Greek Yogurt
17	Scrambled Eggs with Tomato	Zucchini and Tomato Frittata	Tofu and Vegetable Curry	Kiwi Slices
18	Oatmeal with Maple Syrup	Turkey and Quinoa Bowl	Baked Chicken Thighs with Carrots	Rice Crackers with Tzatziki
19	FODMAP-Friendly Banana Bread	Spinach and Feta Omelette	Grilled Shrimp with Quinoa	Lactose-Free Cheese and Grapes
20	Smoothie with Papaya	Low FODMAP Caesar Salad	Egg Fried Rice with Shrimp	Mixed Nuts

21	Greek Yogurt with Raspberries	Chicken and Vegetable Stir-Fry	Baked Cod with Lemon and Dill	Orange Slices with Almond Butter